CONT

This book is presented as a collection of natural remedies and as an aid in understanding their use. It is not intended to replace or supersede professional consultation or treatment and no guarantee can be given as to the efficacy or appropriateness of a remedy in an individual case without professional advice.

INTRODUCTION

S tress has become an unwelcome but accepted part of modern life.

While a certain amount of stress can be considered a good thing – it can supply the adrenalin we sometimes need and can also give us a push towards making changes in our lives – if we're under too much stress, the balance is tipped and unwanted symptoms like anxiety, sleeplessness, headaches or stomach pains may begin to manifest themselves.

Natural remedies and therapies can help greatly in relieving feelings of stress and associated symptoms, and can be an ideal support whilst working towards the only permanent way to reduce the amount of stress in our lives, which is to choose – or find – another way of doing things.

WHY DO WE GET STRESSED?

We may experience some types of short-term stress as a positive thing and even seek it out to give a little excitement to our life.

A feeling of satisfaction and exhilaration may follow the successful completion of an event before which you felt stressed. Examples of this could be a sporting event like running a marathon, or a parachute jump or public speaking.

Many actors say they feel nervous or stressed before a performance, but that they use that energy to give their acting an 'edge' that it would lack without this anticipation. Sometimes these feelings of being under pressure can get out of control, though, and hinder our performance, such as before a driving test or exam, and then it can be helpful to take a natural remedy, such as homœopathic *Arg nit*, which will calm our nerves but not hamper our ability (see Anxiety page 22).

STRESSFUL EVENTS

There are some things that we would all find stressful, because they are difficult or traumatic experiences – such as the death of a loved one, breaking up of a relationship, being made redundant, illness, etc. In these instances we know we need to give ourselves time to recover our equilibrium, and look after ourselves as best we can in the meantime. Natural remedies, such as herbs, can be used to support the nervous system and, for example, aid sleep during such a time (see the Remedies that Really Work section, page 22 onwards).

MULTIPLE FACTORS

At other times there may not be one single event that we can attribute our feelings of being stressed to. We often simply get used to working to tight deadlines, a relationship that is just about ok, commuting to work, supporting the kids/parents financially and emotionally, never getting quite enough sleep, drinking coffee to get through the day, but then one more (not necessarily major) thing comes along and tips the balance.

We may not even realise how much stress we've been carrying, but then start waking at night and going over and over the events of the day – a sure sign that sufficient space and time hasn't been given to process thoughts at a better time – or our bowels start playing up, we experience a panic attack, or our skin breaks out... and we are forced to recognise that we're not coping with the pressures of life as well as we thought. In this instance natural remedies can be used to relieve the symptoms, but it will also be necessary to make some lifestyle changes to reduce the amount of ongoing stress being experienced, and the damaging effect that it is having.

The suggestions in this booklet will help you to find the appropriate remedies to help support you, and also give you some ideas for making the kind of changes that will permanently reduce your stress load, so that you can enjoy life more fully and experience a greater sense of vitality and well-being.

WHEN GOOD STRESS BECOMES BAD

The stress response of the body is there to protect and support us in emergency situations.
To maintain stability or homeostasis, the body is constantly adjusting to its surroundings; when an event threatens this equilibrium, we react to it. This ability to react quickly is a basic survival mechanism, often referred to as the "fight or flight response". We prepare for physical action in order to confront or flee a threat.

THE SURVIVAL MECHANISM

For our ancestors, this survival mechanism would have enabled them to hunt and escape from wild animals and respond to the stressful ordeals of inhabiting a more dangerous world. Millions of years later, when you face a situation that you perceive as challenging, your body automatically goes into overdrive, engaging the same stress response. What happens physically is that you release hormones and your heartbeat speeds up, your blood pressure increases and your breathing quickens; this results in your being able to move and think faster, hit harder, see better, hear more acutely, and jump higher than you could only seconds earlier.

What should follow the surge of energy released following such an event is a period of relaxation so that the body can fully recharge itself, and hopefully also a celebration of having survived (or for a hunter, the satisfaction of having caught a good meal).

What seems to have happened in modern life is that although we rarely have to escape from dangerous animals or hunt for our dinner, we constantly push ourselves on a daily basis; as the saying goes, we expect to 'work hard and play hard'. The kind of ongoing stresses that we experience commonly today are things like: driving in busy traffic, working to tight deadlines, dealing with aggressive behaviour from other people, juggling a busy work schedule with running a house, moving home, caring for children or sick relatives, financial worries, taking exams, etc.

HORMONES

The problem is that the same hormones are released during emotional stress as physical stress, so both will affect each other. Then you actually get used to living with a constant low-level of stress hormones being released all the time. Our expectations of performance become adjusted to being constantly on alert and on a heightened level, and of course other peoples' expectations of us will also tend to reinforce that as our norm.

Eventually, if we don't relax properly and experience feelings of happiness and well-being regularly, the feelings of stress build up in our system and we begin to get symptoms of dis-ease like tiredness, agitation and difficulty switching off when we want to.

To maintain a busy lifestyle we often drink coffee and take other stimulants, until we begin to rely on them 'to get us going in the morning', or keep us working into the evening. We get used to never having quite enough sleep or time to relax and think through our problems.

When we get a headache, instead of going to bed we take a painkiller so that we can keep working. If we get a cold we take an aspirin to suppress the fever and medication to dry up the mucus, so that we can keep going rather than staying at home and nursing ourselves better. Is it any wonder then that at some point our body begins to rebel and show symptoms of needing to be looked after better?

SYMPTOMS OF STRESS

The following symptoms can all be caused, or aggravated, by stress. In fact some experts say that 90% of illness is caused by stress, which shows how essential it is to learn to deal with it better.

- sleep disturbances
- back, shoulder or neck pain
- tension or migraine headaches
- upset or acid stomach, cramps, heartburn, gas, irritable bowel syndrome
- constipation, diarrhoea
- weight gain or loss, eating disorders
- hair loss
- muscle tension
- fatigue
- high blood pressure
- irregular heartbeat, palpitations
- asthma or shortness of breath
- chest pain
- skin problems (hives, eczema, psoriasis, rashes)
- jaw pain
- menstrual problems
- infertility
- sexual difficulties
- immune system suppression: more colds, 'flu, infections
- nervousness, anxiety, panic attacks
- depression, moodiness
- irritability, frustration
- memory problems
- lack of concentration

POST-TRAUMATIC STRESS DISORDER

Post-traumatic stress disorder is a psychiatric disorder that can occur following the experience or witnessing of life-threatening events, such as natural disasters, terrorist incidents, serious accidents, military combat or violent personal assaults like rape. An estimated 10% of women and 5% of men will experience post-traumatic stress disorder at some point in their lives, and this figure increases to 30% for those who spend time in a war zone.

The most commonly experienced symptoms include reliving the experience through nightmares and flashbacks, difficulty sleeping, and feelings of being detached or estranged. Most survivors of a trauma will recover by themselves given a little time, but some people will have symptoms that do not go away on their own, or may even get worse over time, and this is called post-traumatic stress disorder (PTSD).

Psychological therapies have been proven to be of benefit in treating post-traumatic stress disorder, with cognitive-behavioural therapy being especially successful. The organisation Frontline Homeopathy, which provides homœopathic treatment in countries suffering the effects of war, natural disaster and poverty, has also reported excellent response rates to homœopathic treatment in individuals, both immediately following and months or even years after traumatic events.

For first-aid treatment following a traumatic event, see the section on Anxiety on page 22. To treat post-traumatic stress disorder successfully requires professional help from an experienced practitioner, who can combine counselling skills with the appropriate remedies (see the Contacts on page 30).

TURNING THINGS AROUND

It is in the area of stress that we can perhaps see more clearly than in any other the interconnected link between our mind, body and emotions.

We often first register stress as an emotional response, by feeling agitated or being irritable, but we know that stress is also responsible for a wide range of physical symptoms, from stomach problems to skin conditions or an increased likelihood of going down with a cold or 'flu. Being in a stressful situation will trigger a release of hormones that will affect us mentally and emotionally as well as physically, and in a feedback loop, the hormones flowing around our system will make us feel stressed.

Dealing with the symptoms of stress in a solely physical way, such as taking sleeping tablets for insomnia, may get the quickest results in the short term, but it rarely solves the problem for long. The feelings and symptoms of stress are likely to keep returning unless we also look at the underlying factors in our lifestyle that are contributing to the stress, and thus break the cycle.

Because stress affects us as a whole, lasting benefits will only come from tackling the problem on more than one level. If we examine the effects of stress and also take steps to deal positively with stress physically, emotionally and in our creative life (spiritually), we will learn something about how we developed the symptoms we have and also, more importantly, begin to work out the most effective strategies for us as an individual to cure ourselves of the problem.

3 STEPS TO SURVIVING STRESS

When we experience the symptoms of stress, it is an indication that there is an imbalance in our life.

When we become stuck in this imbalance we will begin to display the symptoms of disease.

By considering each of the areas of our lives laid out in the 3 steps below we are able to get some insight into where to begin in making positive changes, and also get suggestions for practical steps to support the areas where help is needed most.

STEP 1 – SUPPORTING YOUR BODY

Long term exposure to the hormones that are released when experiencing stress damages your body. If, as mentioned earlier, 90% of illness can be related back to stress, it shows how imperative it is to reduce the impact of it on your body. Whether you are experiencing stress now, or you have recently been through a period of stress, you need to take steps to repair the damage and build in some reserves to prevent further damage.

NUTRITION – THE BASIC ELEMENTS OF REPAIR

How do you support yourself physically? Firstly, through a good diet. It is impossible to feel fit, healthy and well if you eat a diet based on pre-packaged, chemical laden, mass-produced food that is high in unhealthy fats and sugars and poor in nutrients. What you need is a diet based on fresh – preferably organic – whole foods, full of vitality and rich in the vitamins, minerals and other nutrients that your body needs to continually repair itself. Eating well also makes a positive statement about looking after yourself, especially when a lot is being demanded of you.

Our bodies use up the B group vitamins particularly rapidly when we are under stress and a shortage of these can cause nervous system disorders such as feelings of agitation, increased pain, sleeplessness and also pre-menstrual tension. So it is important to get sufficient B vitamins in your diet, or if that isn't practical, to take a B complex food supplement. Foods naturally rich in B vitamins include: yeast extract, meat, oily fish, eggs, brown rice, wheatgerm, beans, sunflower seeds, nuts.

NATURAL REMEDIES

One of the great benefits of natural remedies is that they support your body's natural healing mechanisms as the way to creating health. The remedies discussed below and in the Remedies that Really Work section will all help to support and strengthen your body as a way of relieving the impact and symptoms of stress.

Try the remedies out – they are included because they are suitable for use by you at home – **although anyone already taking medication should check with a qualified herbalist before taking herbal remedies.** Also, selecting and taking a remedy for yourself is an empowering experience; you have made a positive choice, and you will also learn about a remedy and your response to it.

Herbal De-Stress Blend – Gotu Kola, Damiana, Lemon Balm, Skullcap, Vervain

This is an effective blend of herbs that will support your nervous system and generally relieve common symptoms of stress such as sleeplessness and anxiety. Combine the herbs to make an infusion, or for greater convenience use the tinctures (a liquid preparation of herbs) and take 3 times a day as required. If things are not greatly relieved after a few weeks then try out some of the more specific remedies in the Remedies that Really Work section, or seek professional advice from a qualified herbalist. *This blend is not suitable to take during pregnancy.*

Siberian Ginseng

This is an herb known as an adaptogen, which means it increases the capacity of the body to adapt to and cope with physical and mental stress. Siberian Ginseng is used widely in Russia and has been proven to improve levels of stamina and endurance and also to increase resistance to infectious illnesses such as colds and 'flu. It also promotes the ability of your body to adapt better to environmental stresses such as pollution and various types of radiation damage. Take the tincture 3 times a day for several weeks. It may be taken in conjunction with the De-stress blend above.

When to See a Practitioner

If you try a natural remedy and you don't get much improvement after a few weeks, or sooner if your symptoms are more severe, or if you are suffering with a more serious underlying health problem, then visit a qualified practitioner.

Even those of us who are practitioners can feel stuck with a health problem from time to time, and then it is time to consult someone else and get a different viewpoint and specialised assistance. See the list of Contacts at the back of the booklet to help you find a suitable practitioner or, better still, see someone recommended by a friend or colleague.

There are many therapies that have a good track record of relieving stress symptoms – in particular, aromatherapy massage, homœopathy, acupuncture, medical herbalism and shiatsu.

Rest

Our body needs sufficient rest and sleep to repair itself and stay healthy. Most adults need a minimum of 7 hours of sleep a night on a regular basis to feel good.

Obviously we can get by on less than that, as any parent of young children will know, but that is about what is needed to do more than just survive, and to really allow the body sufficient time to repair and restore itself. So to overcome the symptoms of stress you will need to build into your lifestyle the possibility of at least 7 hours of sleep a night, or a short nap in the day if 7 hours at night isn't achievable.

If sleeplessness is one of the symptoms of stress that you are currently experiencing, then look at the section on page 27 for some strategies and remedies to help you.

Exercise – Proven to Reduce Stress Symptoms

For us to feel good in our body, and for our body to stay fit and healthy, we need to take regular exercise. Moreover, not only is introducing exercise linked to decreased anxiety and depression, but the physically active suffer less from stress and stress – associated illnesses than the non-active – the so called 'stress-buffering' role (Brown, Journal of Personality and Social Psychology, 1991).

There are a number of things that occur during exercise that seem to cause these beneficial effects, including increased release of endorphins (the hormones associated with feeling happy), reduced muscle tension and reduced excitability of the nervous system, as well as the improvement of self-esteem, and, obviously, physical fitness. In fact, Dr Blumenthal, a professor of medical psychology at Duke University claims that, "exercise seems to be at least as effective as standard antidepressant medications in reducing symptoms in patients with depression".

So what kind of exercise is best? In studies, a moderate level of exercise has been shown to be the most beneficial. Too low a level of exercise has little beneficial effect and excessive exercise can actually increase stress levels. Moderate exercise will mean you may become slightly breathless, and you will need to exercise for about 30 minutes a day on most days of the week.

Walking, cycling, swimming, playing sport at a low level, gardening and line dancing have all been shown to be effective for stress management. The important factor is to be active frequently enough, which means 5–6 days a week.

The key is finding a type of exercise that you enjoy enough to do regularly and if you really do not have the time to take out for an activity (if you are a working mother for example), then make sure you take a brisk walk whenever you have the opportunity during the day – to the train station, to get yourself a sandwich at lunchtime, walking up stairs, pushing the pram, etc.

STEP 2 – SUPPORTING YOUR EMOTIONAL BALANCE

It is a combination of the way that we are doing things, our lifestyle, and our response to what's happening in our lives that has led to us getting in a stressed state. So how do we begin to sort this out and become healthier and enjoy ourselves more?

We need to appreciate our life as a process of transformation and growth and we need to look at some of the habits that are preventing that growth.

The ups and downs of daily life will mean that we get to experience a range of emotions, some that we call good and some that we call bad. When we get stuck with a negative feeling, we may begin to recognise this as a symptom of stress.

We may start to get irritable and short-tempered with our loved ones or tearful over trivial things, or begin to feel anxious for no apparent reason or even have a panic attack. Sometimes we simply feel 'not right', but it is hard to define what the problem is. These are all indications that something is blocking our ability to change and grow and adapt joyfully to life's experiences.

Moving on

What we need to do is first acknowledge these feelings, and then treat them as signs that some kind of change is needed. Being happy and healthy is an ongoing process – it is not something that you arrive at, and then that's it for evermore. We have to constantly adapt and grow to meet new challenges.

One of the most powerful things that you can do when things are getting you down is to acknowledge that you are a bit stuck, and seek some help or advice. Making an appointment with a practitioner, whether it is to receive a stress-relieving massage or for a course of counselling sessions, will often make you start to feel better in itself. Taking a positive decision to do something to help yourself is very empowering, and most holistic therapists will be able to help you unravel some of the causes of your stress as well as treat whatever particular symptoms you are experiencing.

Habits

It should be said that changing a habit is easier said than done. However, to break out of a cycle of stress and stop it from returning, finding another way of doing things – choosing to let go of a habit – will be necessary.

Habitual behaviour limits our ability to change and be healthy, and much of it is part of a pattern of fear: fear of change, of disapproval, of being criticised or of not being loved. For example, if I am always busy, rushing around doing things for other people, I can convince myself that I am 'an important person', and not, as I fear, someone who isn't really very significant.

Positive steps

For many people in the modern world gaining a better emotional balance will mean reprioritising, so that more time can be spent on really satisfying things. Time management courses or books can help you to impose a more effective structure on your life, which can be a great antidote to feeling overwhelmed.

When you are feeling really stressed concentrate on doing what is essential to look after yourself and take small steps, try to eat and sleep well, and consider what you can say 'no' to. Try to create a bit of space in your life so that you can reflect on what beneficial changes you can make. There are many opportunities nowadays – such as counselling and life coaching practitioners, and retreats or 'space clearing' workshops – that can be very helpful in supporting you to make positive changes to your lifestyle.

BACH FLOWER REMEDIES

Flower remedies address the mood and emotional outlook of a person, restoring peace of mind and allowing the body to fight illness by strengthening its inner resources. They were first discovered by Dr Bach during the 1930s, and many other ranges have been developed since then. Flower remedies are made by using sunlight to infuse a bowl of water with the essence of various flowers.

The Bach flower remedies work not by attacking disease, but by releasing and strengthening the energy within that inner part of yourself that knows how and what needs healing and which is often hidden by our reaction to life's stresses and difficulties. They are completely safe to take by all, including children and babies, and will not interfere with other treatments or medication. Simply add a few drops to water and take several times a day.

There are 38 individual Bach flower remedies and you can contact the Healing Herbs of Dr Bach for information and literature on the full range. The following blends have been developed by Julian Barnard of the Flower Essence Program and can be mixed yourself by adding each of the individual remedies listed to a dropper bottle. Alternatively, they can be purchased ready-mixed from Neal's Yard Remedies.

To choose a remedy simply read the descriptions below and pick the one that most closely matches your feelings at this moment in time.

Courage

This blend encourages calm control and courage when fears and apprehensions have taken over. It gently dispels fearfulness and inner turmoil so feelings of security and safety can take root.

Indicated for: panic, fears, shyness, trembling, fear for others or the world, fear of hurting self or others, mental torment.

Contains: honeysuckle, cherry plum, mimulus, red chestnut, rock rose, aspen, agrimony.

Confidence & Power

Supports assertiveness and inner strength when life's challenges have sapped motivation and esteem. It brings a stronger sense of individuality & the ability to function with more integrity.

Indicated for: poor sense of self, belittled, apologetic, lacking of confidence, powerless, feeling inferior, submissive, discouraged, self-sacrificing.

Contains: larch, centaury, rock rose, gentian, elm, pine.

Direction

A supporting blend during times of personal transformation when direction may be lost and decision-making is hard. Promotes clarity and increased self-understanding.

Indicated for: lack of commitment, mid-life crisis, career changes, doubt, indecision, apathy, fear of future, lack of responsibility.

Contains: scleranthus, wild oat, cerato, walnut, mimulus, wild rose.

Focus

Helps clear the head and increase confidence in the self, and brings a positive attitude to learning and academic work. It can help focus the mind if under the pressure of deadlines.

Indicated for: exams, interviews, cramming, mental tiredness, overwhelm, fear of failure, revision, feeling distracted and fuzzy-headed, mental chatter, lack of inspiration.

Contains: larch, elm, white chestnut, hornbeam, gentian, clematis.

Letting Go

Promotes acceptance and understanding when anger and bitterness seem uppermost in the mind, and life feels unfair. Could also bring essential insight into the self.

Indicated for: resentment, intolerance, co-dependence, neediness, unhappiness, relationship problems, attention-seeking, blaming, indifference, distancing, a tendency to being controlling and resistance to change.

Contains: holly, willow, vine, beech, chicory, water violet.

Optimism

Brings a renewal of optimism and faith when life feels impossible. It brings about a gentle rebirth as it lifts the self out of intense darkness and into the light.

Indicated for: moodiness, gloom, despondency, adolescence, discouragement, hopelessness, pessimism, despair, dark-night of the soul, loneliness.

Contains: gorse, gentian, mustard, sweet chestnut, cherry plum, heather.

Revitalise

Brings strength and energy when life's responsibilities have taken their toll and fatigue has set in. It helps a depleted system recuperate by making available essential support & vitality.

Indicated for: feeling debilitated, burnt-out, overworked, strained and drained (especially carers), no get up and go, overwhelmed, low, fragile, weak, out of sorts. Also for menstrual stress.

Contains: olive, elm, oak, crab apple, hornbeam, walnut.

Unwind

Brings welcome relief when it becomes increasingly difficult to relax, switch off and recharge with a refreshing night's sleep.

Indicated for: stress, being uptight and overwrought, striving, impatience, perfectionism, worry, restless nights, working too hard.

Contains: vervain, impatiens, agrimony, rock water, walnut, aspen, white chestnut.

S.O.S

Dr Bach's classic rescue combination promotes feelings of calm and serenity and is for life's most extreme challenges or situations. Frequent use is suggested during those times.

Indicated for: emergencies, bereavement, interviews, life dramas, emotional situations, travel, public speaking, exam nerves, anguish.

Contains: clematis, impatiens, rock rose, star of Bethlehem, cherry plum.

STEP 3 – SUPPORTING YOUR SPIRITUAL SELF

It would be rare for every area of our life – family, friends, work, finances, living situation, etc. – to all be working perfectly well at the same time. It is more normal for some things to be going well, and some things to be causing us a bit of concern. However, providing we feel basically on track with our life we can usually cope with the day-to-day problems that life throws up and still feel okay about life as a whole.

The key here is to feel our life is generally heading in the right direction, that there is a central sense of okay-ness about what we are doing. Nearly everyone needs a sense of purpose or direction to experience wellbeing. And if we have that basic feeling, then we are better able to cope with the ups and downs of living without feeling overly stressed. This is one of the main functions of religion – to provide that sense of purpose – and an important reason why people often turn to religion at times of crisis; it can help people to reprioritise their lives.

One of the main problems with feeling stressed is that we tend to lose that sense of direction and feel scattered, overwhelmed or pulled in too many different directions. When that happens we lose touch with that positive feeling of being on track and centred. It becomes difficult to take satisfaction in what we do achieve each day, and we are then likely to experience symptoms such as anxiety, insomnia and stomach problems that are associated with being stressed.

Nearly all of us will recognise the experience of feeling in contact with something greater than ourselves at some time in our lives, and the aim of cultivating our spiritual life is to have constant access to this source of energy, to get it flowing through every aspect of our lives. It is this impersonal love that brings the gift of enjoyment and wellbeing into our lives.

How Do I Support My Spiritual Self?

It is essential to recognise that we do have a spiritual side to our lives that needs to be nurtured, just as our physical body does. The spiritual side of our life is that inner sense of self and creative energy that keeps us motivated and growing as people, and it requires us to be actively engaged in the process known as 'becoming conscious'.

This means being constantly willing to think about what we do and how we live, examining all our old patterns and habits and opening up to life as a process of insight, inspiration and purposefulness.

We may not all be lucky enough to have a job that we feel is a true expression of our inner purpose, but we can all make sure that we do something regularly that we find to be totally satisfying and creative. If nothing springs to mind then think about what you really enjoyed doing as a child – was it painting or playing in the garden, learning a new skill or looking after a pet? Then apply that to your adult life and get back into painting, pottery, or experiencing nature... maybe take a course in gardening, natural medicine, or whatever attracts you.

If you are feeling lost and uncertain as to what direction to take in life then the Bach flower blend called Direction will help to promote clarity, self-understanding and decision-making during times of doubt and uncertainty. It contains a combination of scleranthus, wild oat, cerato, walnut, mimulus and wild rose. Simply take a few drops in water several times a day.

We need to reassess our lives regularly to check that our lifestyle is still supporting our inner purpose, and question whether we are avoiding what we really feel we should be doing with our life by getting caught up in rushing around, drinking alcohol, taking drugs, gathering possessions and interacting superficially with people.

Being healthy spiritually means building in time to reflect on where our life is going. It also means being prepared to accept symptoms, such as those caused by stress, as signs that we are not 'on track' and that we may need to adjust or change something about the way we are living.

MEDITATION

Meditation is a powerful tool that has been taught by many spiritual traditions to calm the chattering of our brain, and create a contact with the part of our mind that uses symbols and images, and is beyond the rational and mundane. Meditation can help us to restore our contact with ourselves, and with our real needs, so that we are motivated from inside and not constantly subject to what happens to us from the outside and reacting to our environment.

BENEFITS OF MEDITATION FOR REDUCING STRESS

Scientific studies overwhelmingly support meditation practice to reduce stress, recover from or prevent certain diseases, and improve overall health. One such study, at the University of Massachusetts Mindfulness Stress Reduction Program, included positive results from over 13,000 people. Other research studies indicate that people who practice some form of meditation outlive those people who do not (Time Magazine, The Science of Meditation, 2003).

Herbert Benson, a Harvard cardiologist, conducted research that showed a variety of different types of meditation produced what he called the 'relaxation response'. This response includes a significant decrease in the levels of cortisol and other stress hormones within the body, as well as generating calmer breathing and heart rate, a decline in blood pressure and relaxation of muscles. Moreover, in 2005 researchers at Yale University used MRIs to scan the brains of 20 people who meditate daily, comparing their brains to a group of people who did not meditate.

The scans showed that the meditators had thicker grey matter in the cerebral cortex and in an area of the brain linked to emotions and attention. These were ordinary people with jobs and families. The researcher Jeremy Gray observed, "Daily meditation actually creates physical changes in the brain, growing new cells in regions responsible for concentration and making sense of the world".

Specifically with regard to stress reduction, researchers from West Virginia University carried out a study of 62 stressed people, which involved an 8-week course where participants learnt 4 types of meditation, some basic yoga postures and how to use meditation in their normal lives once the course had finished. Results showed over half the subjects experienced a drop in psychological distress, by an average of 54%. The study also showed a 46% drop in the medical symptoms they had experienced as a result of stress (American Journal of Health Promotion, July 2001).

Studies have also been done that show how meditation can decrease stress in the workplace. One 3 month study of managers and employees (of one large and one smaller company in the USA) who regularly practiced meditation, showed that meditation practitioners displayed more relaxed physiological functioning, greater reduction in anxiety, and reduced tension on the job, when compared to control subjects with similar job positions in the same companies (Anxiety, Stress and Coping International Journal, 6, 1993).

WHAT KIND OF MEDITATION IS BEST?

There are lots of different kinds of meditation, some concentrating more on breathing, others on imaging, some using a word repeated over and over (mantra), others combined with exercise (certain types of yoga).

What they have in common is that they calm the active, 'chattering' part of the mind and connect us to an experience of ourselves that is beyond that of the petty personality, and linked to our source of joy, and feeling of true connection with the universe and our inner strength.

There is no such thing as the best type of meditation, only the one that suits you best – you may need to try 2 or 3 different types of meditation before you find the one that feels totally right for you. It is similar to finding the best kind of exercise; the essential thing is to choose one that you can build into your lifestyle and do regularly.

There are many books, leaflets, adverts, cd's, websites, etc. promoting various kinds of meditation available these days. You could start by finding out which groups meet nearby e.g. in your nearest natural therapy centre, or look in a good 'alternative' bookshop for a cd or book if you would prefer to try it alone. Probably best of all is to ask people you respect if they have ever done any kind of meditation and how they got on with it.

SOME COMMON PROBLEMS & REMEDIES THAT REALLY WORK

The following remedies are all tried and tested for treating the symptoms of stress. Try them out for a while and see if you get relief. If they don't seem to work and new symptoms develop or symptoms keep returning seek professional advice. Anyone already taking medication should see a herbalist before taking a new herbal remedy.

ANXIETY (AND PANIC ATTACKS)

Feelings of anxiety can be an early indicator of stress. Anxiety is recognised by a feeling of uneasiness and apprehension accompanied with tension, which may be associated with tight breathing, palpitations and perspiration.

A full blown panic attack may appear to come 'out of the blue' but is nearly always directly related to going through a stressful time, and is best treated by taking emergency remedies described below (Aconite, S.O.S.) during the attack, and then taking remedies to support and calm the nervous system along with steps to deal with stress in the longer term.

Diet, as always, has an important role to play. Check especially that your diet contains sufficient calcium and magnesium, and vitamins B and C, or if in doubt take a multivitamin and mineral supplement.

The following remedies will help relieve the symptoms, but if the anxiety is extreme a qualified practitioner should be consulted. You can combine some of the suggestions below – for example, take the herbal tea blend in conjunction with the most appropriate homœopathic remedy.

HERBS FOR ANXIETY

Chamomile, Lemon Balm, Passiflora, Scullcap, Valerian, Vervain

These herbs will all soothe stress, relieve feelings of anxiety and panic, and strengthen the nervous system. Combine and drink a cupful of infusion, or take as a tincture blend, three times a day. Omit the vervain during pregnancy.

HOMŒOPATHY FOR ANXIETY

Aconite 30

Anxiety dating from a fright, shock or accident. Panic attacks with fear of imminent death. One dose twice a day for 2 or 3 days.

Arg Nit 30

Anxiety and apprehension before an event – exam, flight, public speaking, etc. Anticipatory diarrhoea. One or two doses.

Ignatia 30

Anxiety dating from a particular emotional disappointment such as a relationship breakdown, bereavement, etc. Take one dose each evening for a week.

ESSENTIAL OILS FOR ANXIETY

Geranium, Lavender, Neroli, Orange, Ylang Ylang

Combine 2 or 3 of these oils and dilute in a bath oil base to add to the bath, or dilute in a suitable base massage oil for a calming massage.

BACH FLOWER REMEDIES FOR ANXIETY

S.O.S

Dr Bach's classic rescue combination promotes feelings of calm and serenity and is for life's most extreme challenges and situations. It will relieve symptoms of anxiety, and panic attacks, and can be used for accidents, interviews, life dramas, emotionally fraught situations, travel or exam nerves, etc. Frequent use is suggested during those times. It contains clematis, impatiens, rock rose, star of Bethlehem and cherry plum.

Unwind

Brings welcome relief to symptoms of anxiety and agitation when accompanied by feelings of stress, impatience, worry, and being overwrought, over-worked and sleepless. It will promote the ability to relax, switch off and recharge with a refreshing night's sleep. It is a combination of vervain, impatiens, agrimony, rock water, walnut, aspen and white chestnut.

FATIGUE (AND POOR LIBIDO)

One response to stress is to feel low in energy and weary or depressed. This lack of energy often extends to a loss of interest in sex and poor libido. (Obviously if fatigue is severe or prolonged then you should seek professional advice to rule out any underlying health problem.) There are some excellent natural remedies that act as tonics to support and strengthen your resources.

A good diet will be essential in restoring energy and vitality. If in doubt take a multivitamin and mineral supplement. The iron supplement Floradix can be helpful if you suspect anaemia may be involved.

HERBS FOR FATIGUE

Alfalfa, Lemon Balm, Nettle, Vervain

These herbs will nourish your body, gently strengthen and support your nervous system and lift your spirits. Combine and make an infusion to drink 3 times a day or take the tinctures. *Omit the vervain during pregnancy.*

Damiana

Add this aphrodisiac and antidepressant herb to the above mixture to boost your general vitality and libido if you are also suffering with low spirits or a poor sex drive. Suitable for men and women.

Ginseng

An excellent general tonic that has been used for thousands of years in China to strengthen reserves of energy and resistance to stress. Ginseng also acts as an effective aphrodisiac for poor libido. Best taken as a tincture 3 times a day. Do not take during pregnancy, if you suffer with high blood pressure or when you have a fever such as when suffering a cold or 'flu.

Essential Oils for Fatigue

Geranium, Grapefruit, Frankincense, Lavender, Rosemary

Choose 2 or 3 of the oils and dilute in a vegetable oil base to add to the bath or for massage. May also be used in a burner or diffuser.

Bach Flower Remedies for Fatigue

Revitalise

Brings strength and energy when life's responsibilities have taken their toll and fatigue has set in. This blend helps a depleted system recuperate by making available essential support and vitality. It contains olive, elm, oak, crab apple, hornbeam and walnut.

HEADACHES

Tension headaches are a common symptom of stress and can be relieved by natural remedies – although if they recur frequently, then some of the steps described earlier to reduce stress will need to be taken in addition to the recommendations here.

The simplest treatment for a tension headache is to drink plenty of water (many headaches are caused by dehydration) and get some rest; often what is required is an early night and not medication.

Migraine headaches are a particularly intense type of headache; often accompanied by vision disorders and nausea. The pain is caused by a spasm of blood vessels in the brain. Best results will be achieved by visiting a qualified practitioner for constitutional treatment. The causes of migraine can be complex and varied although many sufferers obtain relief if they reduce the stress levels in their life, and high stress is often a contributory factor in the frequency of attacks.

If headaches are very severe or persistent, or are caused by injury, immediate medical treatment must be sought.

Herbs for Headaches

Chamomile, Lemon Balm, Peppermint, Rosemary, Vervain

Combine the herbs and make an infusion to drink every 4 hours, or use the tinctures. During pregnancy only chamomile and lemon balm may be taken.

Feverfew

Research has shown that this anti-inflammatory herb can be very effective at preventing migraine in a significant number of sufferers. Best taken as capsules on a regular basis until the condition is stabilised, and then take at the first sign of symptoms. *Not suitable for use during pregnancy.*

HOMŒOPATHY FOR HEADACHES

Belladonna 30

Throbbing headache. Head may feel congested or hot. One dose every 2 hours.

Bryonia 30

Bursting, heavy, crushing headache that is worse for any movement and relieved by lying still. May be associated with feeling thirsty or constipated. One dose every 4 hours.

Gelsemium 30

Heavy, dull headache. Eyelids feel droopy. Often associated with other 'flu-like symptoms. May be caused by anticipation before a stressful event. One dose every 4 hours.

Nux vomica 30

Headache associated with feeling irritable. May be brought on by overindulgence in stimulants (alcohol, coffee, cigarettes, etc.) – known as the hangover cure. Can also be brought on by over-concentrating. Often accompanied by nausea. One dose every 4 hours.

ESSENTIAL OILS FOR HEADACHES

Bergamot, Lavender, Rosemary, Peppermint

Choose one or two oils and dilute in a vegetable oil base to add to the bath, or to massage into the feet and draw tension away from the head.

Lavender

Apply one drop to each temple to bring relief.

INSOMNIA

Most people will suffer with the odd sleepless night at some time. It can, though, become rather a habit and then anxiety can develop around not being able to sleep. In other words, stress can cause sleeplessness and then not getting enough sleep contributes to feelings of stress, and a vicious cycle is set up.

The following remedies will help to break the habit and encourage a good night's sleep, but for chronic insomniacs careful constitutional treatment by a qualified therapist will be necessary.

Sleep disorders such as early morning waking, if accompanied by dark moods, can indicate underlying depression, which may require professional help.

Avoid tea, coffee and other stimulants in the evening if you suffer from sleeplessness – instead replace them with some of the herbal infusions below. Similarly, try to avoid things that are intellectually stimulating or potentially stressful towards bedtime. Physical exercise improves one's ability to sleep soundly, and a daily exercise routine can make a marked difference.

Meditation and visualisation exercises can be used to distract an over-active brain from going round in circles and preventing sleep. Try concentrating on relaxing the entire body, muscle by muscle, from the feet upwards, or running through the events of the day backwards without becoming attached to any one thing in particular.

In summary if you are suffering with a bout of sleeplessness, best results will probably come from a combination of things, such as taking exercise in the day, drinking a herbal infusion in the evening followed by a warm bath with essential oils, then taking the indicated homœopathic or Bach flower remedy and using a visualisation technique when in bed to calm the brain.

HERBS FOR INSOMNIA

Chamomile, Lemon Balm, Lime Flowers, Orange Blossom, Passiflora

A calming and mildly sedative tea to drink in the evening. Make an infusion by adding a heaped teaspoonful of herb mixture to a cupful of boiling water and leaving to infuse for 10 minutes before straining and drinking. Or add the tinctures to hot water.

Vervain, Skullcap

Add these if symptoms of anxiety and tension are marked.
Not suitable to take during pregnancy.

Valerian

This is a very effective sedative herb that may be added to the above mixture or taken on its own for a few days at a time, but it should not be taken long term as it may become habit forming. Best taken as a tincture.

FURTHER READING

Curtis, S., Essential Oils, Haldane Mason

Curtis & Fraser, Natural Healing for Women, Thorsons

Sutton, Annabel, 52 Ways to Handle It – A Lifecoaching Year, Winter Press

Harper-Deacon, J., Meditation CD

CONTACTS

Use these contacts to find a practitioner near you.

HOMŒOPATHY

The Society of Homeopaths
11 Brookfield,
Duncan Close,
Moulton Park,
Northampton
NN3 6WL
Tel: 0845 450 6611
www.homeopathy-soh.org

Alliance of Registered Homeopaths
Millbrook,
Millbrook Hill,
Nutley,
East Sussex
TN22 3PJ
Tel: 08700 736339
www.a-r-h.org

HERBALISM

The National Institute of Medical Herbalists
56 Longbrook Street,
Exeter,
Devon
EX4 6AH
Tel: 01392 426022
www.nimh.org.uk

NUTRITION

British Association for Nutritional Therapy (BANT)
27 Old Gloucester Street,
London
WC1N 3XX
Tel: 0870 606 1284
www.bant.org.uk

SUPPLIERS

NEAL'S YARD REMEDIES

To find your nearest shop contact 01747 834634
Mail order: 0845 262 3145
www.nealsyardremedies.com
- Bach flower essences, herbs, homœopathic remedies, supplements, and natural skin care.
- Therapy rooms offering a wide range of therapies for physical and emotional issues.

AINSWORTH'S HOMŒOPATHIC PHARMACY

36 New Cavendish Street,
London
W1G 8UF
Tel: 020 7935 5330
www.ainsworths.com
Helios Homœopathy

HELIOS HOMŒOPATHY

89-97 Camden Road,
Tunbridge Wells,
Kent
TN1 2QR
www.helios.co.uk
Tel: 01892 537254

PERSONAL NOTES: